YOUR
STRESS
STOPS
HERE!

10 Strategies To Change
Your Habits In
59 Seconds Or Less

Vincent Woon

First Edition 2016

Printed in the United States of America

Published by:

WOON PUBLISHING
1533 13th Street
Fort Lee, NJ 07024

http://www.YourStressStopsHere.com/

For more information about Vincent Woon or to book him for your podcast or media interview please visit: www.StressedOutStressFree.com

Dedication

To my wife Angela for your encouragement and support
and my kids David, Eric, and Joie for your love
and understanding!

Table of Contents

How To Get The Most Out Of This Book

In order for this book to be helpful or useful to you, you must:

- Start with implementing it - take action (without this, nothing works).

- You need to download a *mindfulness app or a reminder app* to act as a reminder throughout your busy schedule to *use these strategies for stress release.* You can set it up every *50 minutes, every hour, 8 times or more a day* (depending on your work hours) when you're at work or whatever time works for you and your schedule. Ideally, you should set it up to remind you once every hour. You'll slowly *integrate these strategies into your life,* and it will eventually *become part of your lifestyle.*

Your stress stops here! You can use any of the strategies in this book to help relieve stress. With the help of the mindfulness bell, or any reminder app, take a break to use these strategies every hour when you are at work or when you are in a stressful situation. Download **Your Stress Stops Here! Journal,** and make sure you record your progress and share it in

our private Facebook group. **To receive your journal and bonus you need to email your receipt to**
join-stress@0s4.com

I recommend the following mindfulness sites and apps:

Popular Websites:

- The Fungie Mindfullness Bell - http://fungie.info/bell/#

- Mindful Clock - http://www.mindfulnessdc.org/mindfulclock.html

Popular phone apps:

- Insight Timer - https://www.InsightTimer.com. It's free and works for iphones and androids.

- Lotus Bud Mindfulness Bell - https://itunes.apple.com/us/app/lotus-bud-mindfulness-bell/id502329366?mt=8 It's free and works for iphones.

- Re.minder - https://itunes.apple.com/us/app/re.minder/id395529341?mt=8. It's free and works for iphones/

After you read each strategy - go ahead and watch the video to see how it's done, use it on yourself, and record it in *Your Stress Stops Here! Journal*. The links are at the end of every strategy.

Note: You ONLY need to sign up once in order to access the video and journal.

ENJOY!

My Background

I am originally from Malaysia. I came to New York in 1983 looking for the American dream. My parents gave me $10,000 for college, and I was on my own for the rest of my school years. My first job was selling Army navy surplus for $30 a day. Later, I found a restaurant job, started working as a busboy, and was promoted to a waiter to help me through college. There was one waitress at the restaurant who liked to give me massages and would ask me to do the same to her. She would always compliment me after I would massage her.

The day after Labor Day, September, 1985, all I remember was riding my bike to school, and the next thing I knew, I was covered under a white cloth, felt pain all over, heard people talking, and I felt like someone was poking something on the top back of the right side of my skull. When I opened my eyes, there were about ten doctors surrounding me. A few of them were tying the stitches on the top right side of my skull.

I was told that I was hit by a delivery truck on Horace Harding expressway, which was only a quarter of my route to school while riding my bicycle. They told me I had fractured my right fibula and tibia (that's both the bones below my knee), a hairline fracture on my pelvis, a broken front tooth, and a big crack on the right side of my head (which they had just finished stitching). Now, that explains the pain I had!

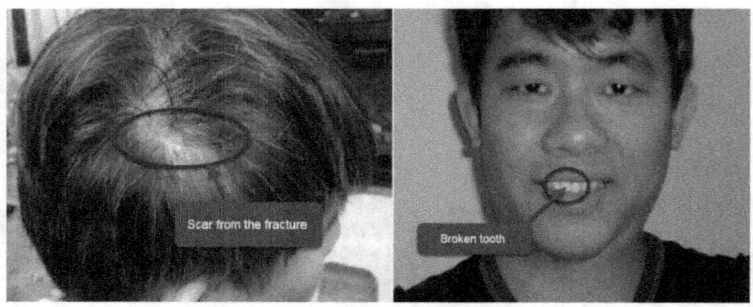

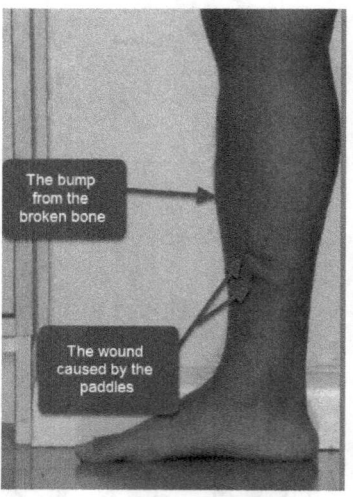

My right leg was in a cast all the way to my mid-thigh with a 4 by 5 opening 3 inches above my ankle for the wound caused by the impact from the bicycle paddle, my pelvis was in a sling, the nerves of my broken front tooth (I had a root canal done on this tooth but it fell off a few years ago and I had to put a bridge over it) were dangling, and I don't know how many stitches I had on my head.

The Weekend Before The Accident

My second sister was getting married that weekend. My eldest sister flew in from Bahrain, my oldest brother flew in from Malaysia to attend the wedding, and my parents and the rest of the family were in Malaysia. My oldest brother and sister were the first people who came to the hospital because they were the only relatives I had around at that time because my second sister left the day before for her honeymoon. My brother in-law flew in from Bahrain with a briefcase full of cash fearing that I wouldn't be able to pay for the medical bill. It's good to have family with you at time like that. I didn't have to pay a single penny for the hospitalization and other rehab; thank God for the no fault insurance law in New York. The total medical bill came out to about sixty thousand dollars for about 2 weeks in the hospital, excluding rehab!

Who's Your Friend?

The first two days in the hospital (in the ICU intensive care unit) were scary because I had to lay in bed with a sling holding my pelvis for the hairline fracture. Every time I moved, I felt aches and pains, and the nerves dangling from my broken tooth were killing me. Every time I closed my mouth, tried to eat, or accidentally touched the nerve with my tongue, it hurt like pouring saline over an open wound. The doctor finally killed the nerve on the third day, which was a major relief for me. My pastor from church came and prayed for me. After the prayer, the fear was gone. My friends came to visit me, and at one point, there were ten of them in my room. There was only two passes per room, but they managed to sneak into my room. Sometimes, it takes something like this to find out who your true friends are. They brought me books to read and food to eat. My friend from work actually gave me a haircut while I was lying down on the bed with my pelvis hanging in a sling at the hospital...that's what you call a friend.

Do You Believe In Angels?

On the fourth day, a lady came to visit me. She introduced herself and told me she was at the scene and had to check with the police to track me down. She came to my rescue and was the one that called the police and got the ambulance to come. She found me on the other side of the road and told me that the opening on my head was pretty big and was bleeding a lot (my wife always make fun of me when I forget something by saying maybe part of my brain fell out at the accident). The lady thought I wouldn't survive, judging from the opening and bleeding on my head. She lost her appetite for the next two days. I would have bleed to death, if it wasn't for her my God sent angel. If not for her, I might not be writing today.

Sometimes people ask me why I believe in Christianity, and my answer to them is Christianity is not a religion; it's a relationship between you and God. I personally experienced God's miracle in my life. By experience, it does not mean you have to get into an accident. It can be an experience that God touched you deeply or maybe you experiences a total change in your life. All you need to do is *believe…that is it!*

Life Goes On

I had to walk around with the cast and crutches for four weeks (that's the time for the bones on my right foot to fully heal) after being discharged from the hospital. I remembered going to Madison Square Garden for bowling, went to the movies, shopping, up and down the subway like what I would normally do. I didn't let the cast and crutches hold me back. You would not notice anything wrong with my foot if you saw me walk. The orthopedic took off the cast on the fourth week, and it was a big relief for me because of the itchiness caused by dryness and sweat.

After taking off the cast, the itchiness was gone, but I still had to learn how to walk again. I had physical therapy three times a week for almost two months. The physical therapist helped me gain my mobility and flexibility. He put my leg into a whirlpool (water reduces stress on the leg) and gave me exercises to strengthen my leg. I had to learn how to use a cane, and later on, my leg was put into a plastic cast to hold it. This enabled me to walk without any support.

My lower back began to give me pain and discomfort, so I bought a massage chair to help me with my back. The chair had not only been a great help to me, but it also became one of my parents' best friends when they were living with me. The massage by the massage chair wasn't as perfect as a massage done by a person, but it provides 75% of my needs.

I went back to school after taking a semester off. I finished college and began working in corporate America. I started working as a temp. Later on, I was promoted to supervisor in the accounting department at a local ethnic newspaper. I enjoyed working there and didn't mind staying late if I had to. All the employees, except for the management staff, were under a union contract and their work hours were 9 to 5.

I worked at the company for five years. The amount of time I spent sitting at the desk in front of the computer, and the amount of stress from all the deadlines for reports and financial statements had put a toll on my body.

I began to feel a constant discomfort on my neck. I always felt like I needed to have my neck adjusted or needed to just pop it, like the way a chiropractor does. My shoulders became tight and always felt like someone was pinching my neck. My lower back hurt, but I didn't understand why. I began to blame all the pain and discomforts on the accident. I was thinking that maybe the accident did something to my neck and shoulder. I must have bumped into something when I was hit by the truck, which threw me across the other side of the road. I was thinking that maybe the hairline fracture caused the pain on my lower back.

I would always find ways, or tried inventing ways, to ease these pains. I constantly stretched and rubbed my shoulder to relieve the pain. After stretching and rubbing my shoulder, I'd try to pop my neck. I would try to twist my back (trying to swing my torso halfway) to release the back pain. I was doing these stretches and twisting so much that my friends were imitating my actions in a game of charades that we played at church. I would ask my wife to stand on my back and lightly jump on it (to crack/pop my back), with me lying face down, to release the stress on my back.

I went to a chiropractor and got a series of treatments and a few adjustments, but it didn't get rid of the pain. In the quest of looking for ways to get rid of these pain and discomfort, I decided to learn massage to help myself. I was also considering a career change because I was tired of the corporate politics. I was going to school again, but this time I felt like I was going to medical school. I had to learn anatomy and physiology while going to work. Learning all the muscles, their origin and attachments, and their actions was quite a challenge, but also fun. It also made me understand why I have the neck pains, shoulder discomfort, and pain on my lower back.

Your Posture Is Important

Looking back, I now realize that the way I sat, the chair I sat on, and my posture made a difference in how I felt. Slowly, I began to use what I've learned in my everyday life. I was able to know how to prevent the pain and also to get rid of the pain. It made me understand where all the tension and pain came from and what I did to cause them to happen. Going to massage school has helped me a lot on my quest of looking for ways to get rid of the pain, but I couldn't keep the stress of politics away. I began to look for a job as a massage therapist upon graduating massage school and getting my license.

My first job as a massage therapist was at a chiropractor's office. It was pretty exciting in the beginning, until later on when he wanted me to do the impossible. The chiropractor wanted me to work on four people 15 minutes each per hour, which was pushing it because I had to allow time for the patient to get ready. After each patient, I have to make sure I have the massage table cleaned and sanitized for the next person while not forgetting the treatment note for every patient.

He bought an aqua massage machine a few months later and wanted me to keep up with the four patients an hour, plus operating the machine. I did my best, but after a month, he fired me. That was the best "fired" I ever had in my life. I thank God for that because if it wasn't for that, I wouldn't have gone and figured it out by my own.

New Discovery

I then worked in health clubs. Later on, I ran a corporate massage program for a company where I would show up twice a week at the company and give massages to all their employees who signed up. I saw, and get to work on, almost everyone in the company from the executives, secretaries, VPs, managers to janitors, IT people, salespeople, receptionists and even the guards.

I began to see how pain or discomfort came from stress at the workplace and how it was affecting them. I was able to incorporate the techniques I used on myself when I was in corporate America, plus what I'd learned in different courses, massage school, and most of all, the different lesson learned from my clients to help relieve the stress of the employees at this company. In addition to that, I saw my own private clients. I have been doing this for the past 20 years.

What's Next

In *Your Stress Stops Here*, I am going to share with you ten of the strategies that I've learned, modified, and improved to meet my needs and your needs to release stress. Use these strategies and slowly turn them into habits to create a stress free lifestyle. I know you'll find these strategies helpful once you implement them and on your way to a stress free lifestyle. To make it easier for you, I've created a journal for you to record your finding from these strategies. When you are finished with the book and journal, you can share it in my private Facebook group.

Thank You and Be Well!

Go ahead and **email your receipt from Amazon to the email below now** to see how it's done. Download *Your Stress Stops Here! Journal* so that you can keep a good record and see your progress.

Email your Amazon Receipt To:
join-stress@0s4.com

CHAPTER 1

A Little Bit About Stress

"Slow down and everything you are chasing will come around and catch you."

- John De Paola

S tress, according to Oxford dictionary, is: A state of mental or emotional strain or tension resulting from adverse or very demanding circumstances. The synonyms for stress are *nervous tension, worry, anxiety, trouble, difficulty, or informal hassle.*

Stress is when you *feel discomfort* even when you sit down, when your *thoughts are running wild.* You feel tension in your body, time pressure holding you back, don't know where to release or direct your energy, and have *difficulty concentrating.* It could be subjected to various *types of demands,* whether physical, mental, or emotional. Contrary to what most people believe, stress is not associated with the negative only since *excessive positive emotions* can result in stress as well. When something that takes place or is about to take place in the environment is producing stress in a person's body, it results into the release of certain chemicals into the bloodstream.

On the positive side, these chemicals can be utilized to *produce more energy* or added strength. This is helpful when the cause of your stress is something physical. However, when you are dealing with emotional stress, it can cause a negative effect on your body, since there is no outlet for releasing that *extra boost of energy and strength*. Therefore, stress results in various *types of emotional or physical responses* because each individual's *body responds differently to the stimulus*. This is also known as fight and flight response, and it's a way your body is protecting you. Some examples would be outrunning a man who jumped in front of you with a knife asking for money, running into a burning building to help save people who's trapped, giving a presentation in front of a hundred people, or meeting someone new.

Whether you admit it or not, stress is a part of everyday life. Whether you are at school, at the office, or just about anywhere, you are forced to deal with people and the environment. Hence, the different types of stress are closely associated with their causes. Because your physical body is *closely connected to your emotional and mental state*, you will notice some connection to their effects when you begin to experience stress. This is the reason why it is important to combat the cause of stress since it affects several vital aspects of your body in order to function.

Types and Causes of Stress

■ *Eustress Stress*[1]

Eustress stress is good stress that motivates you, help you focus your energy, it is short term, is perceived as within your coping abilities, leaves you feeling excited, and improves performance.

---

[1] "Types of Stressors (Eustress vs. Distress) - Mental Help Net." 2015.
    <https://www.mentalhelp.net/articles/types-of-stressors-eustress-vs-distress/>

Examples of Eustress:

- Receiving a promotion.
- Starting a new job.
- Getting married.
- Buying a new home.
- Birth of your child.

■ **Distress Stress**

Distress stress is the unfavorable or negative stress that causes anxiety or concern, can be short or long term, is perceived as outside your coping abilities, feels unpleasant, decreases your performance, and can lead to mental and physical problems.

There are two kinds of distress:

■ ***Acute Stress which arise and quite intense and quickly disappears[2].***

Example of acute stress:

- You have a deadline approaching and stress helps you to focus and finish it before the deadline.
- An accident that crushes your rear bumper.
- Having a problem at work.
- Receiving a phone call from your children's school.
- Running late for work.
- College student cramming to complete project or studying for an exam.

---

[2] "Acute Stress vs. Chronic Stress - Stress - Anxiety." 2008. <http://www.healthcentral.com/anxiety/c/22705/31980/stress-chronic/>

■ *Chronic Stress may not appear quite intense but will linger for a long time.*

Examples of chronic stress:

- Illness in the family.
- Filing a divorce.
- Unemployment.
- Sleep problems.
- Bankruptcy / money problems.
- Separation from a spouse.
- Skin condition like eczema.
- Death of a spouse.
- Death of a family member.

Signs and Symptoms Of Stress[3]

- Muscular tension.
- Constant Headaches.
- High blood pressure.
- Asthma.
- Constant worrying.
- Easily irritable.
- No sex drive.
- Decrease or increase appetite.
- Nausea.
- Constipation.
- Problem sleeping.
- Excessive sweating.
- Teeth grinding.
- Hair loss.
- Reduce immunity.
- Heartburn.

Your stress stops here! You can use any of the strategies in this book at to help relieve stress. With the help of the mindfulness bell, or any reminder app, take a break to use these strategies every hour when you are at work or when you are in a stressful situation.

---

[3] "Stress Effects - American Institute of Stress." 2012. <http://www.stress.org/stress-effects/>

Email your receipt from Amazon to the email below now. Download *Your Stress Stops Here! Journal* so that you can keep a good record and see your progress.

Email your Amazon Receipt To:
join-stress@0s4.com

CHAPTER 2

How Stress
Affect Your Body

---

*"Life is 10% what you experience
and 90% how you respond to it."*

- *Dorothy M. Neddermeyer*

It is important to understand stress and know how it affects your body. In our daily life, we are faced with   frustration, deadlines, and demands, and we become used to stress as if it's part of daily life. A little stress is good, but when it comes to excessive stress, it will turn around and be harmful to us. If it is not addressed, it might even bring death. Let's take a look at what excessive stress can do to your body!

Muscular System

When you are stressed, your muscles begin to contract/tense up; this is called a reflex reaction. The tension or tightness may cause a tension headache or migraine headache, which is normally in head, neck, and shoulder. Past injuries, such as whiplash from a car accident, a fall when you were younger, or even physical abuse, will stress the muscles. Increased tension in your muscle during fight or flight reacts to demand and pressure. Tense muscles get set from reactions to threats and danger. You tend to move faster and have more energy during times of stress. A muscle can go through tension and relaxation indefinitely, but if you do not take the time out to do some relaxation, it will cause the muscle to spasm and cause pain.

The ideal way to achieve muscular relief is to get a massage when you are stressed. You may find it difficult to schedule a massage or might want to put off a massage because of the never ending work in the office and having to take care of your children's schedule of activities (soccer, dance, music, or tennis classes). Most of my clients tended to put off taking care of themselves and put their family first. They didn't realized that if they did not take care of themselves first, they might not be able to take care of their family when they were completely stressed out.

You may sometimes be overwhelmed with work and family activities, but make taking care of yourself a priority because it you don't take care of yourself, how can you take care of the family? Picture this, if you are stressed out, you might be irritated, forgetful, anxious, and hostile when comes to your family activities. These will definitely affect your work and also the life of your family, too. I have seen many of these cases in my practice and came out with ten strategies to help my clients and you to avoid the later. It is important for you to take 59 seconds from every hour out of your busy schedule to do at least one of the ten strategies I am going to show you in the following chapters. Don't forget to download the mindfulness bell, the journal, and join the private Facebook page to share your results with the community. I will have the links at the end of every chapter in all the ten strategies.

Respiratory System

The respiratory system is usually the last thing you are aware of during acute stress because breathing a little faster sometimes seems normal for us. Acute stress is the way the body responds to fight and flight; the body prepares itself for an emergency. When the lungs bring in more oxygen to your body, your blood flow will increase 300 to 400 percent in situations like this. It brings oxygen through the rest of the body by the heart increasing its heart rate. Acute stress can create difficulty for people with asthma or anyone with lung disease.

Cardiovascular System[4]

Emotional and physical stress have negative impacts on the cardiovascular system. Stress is the way your body responds to threats. If the emotional and physical stress continues to repeat itself, it will cause inflammation of the coronary artery and possibly lead to a heart attack.

People with stress appear to have high levels of cholesterol. If not taken care of through medication, diet, or exercise, fat deposits may continue to block the artery wall and may cause a heart attack or stroke. Repeatedly arousing the body's stress increases the blood pressure which damages the heart, blood vessels, and other organs. It also increases the chances of developing a heart disease.

Endocrine System[5]

When stress occurs, your brain will send message to your adrenal gland to release epinephrine, also known as adrenaline, and norepinephrine or noradrenaline into your body. The epinephrine, or adrenaline, rapidly responds by increasing your

---

[4] "How does stress affect cardiovascular health? - AskDoctorK ..." 2012. <http://www.askdoctork.com/how-does-stress-affect-cardiovascular-health-201206292152>

[5] "The Effects of Anxiety on the Endocrine System - Calm Clinic." 2010. <http://www.calmclinic.com/anxiety/symptoms/endocrine-system>

heart rate to pump blood to the muscles and brain. This turns fat into energy, and increases the amount of oxygen to your heart, brain, and muscle to prepare your body to be ready to fight or to flight and be safe.

Epinephrine, or adrenaline, and norepinephrine, or noradrenaline, together with other hormones from almost every organ are released when you are stressed. The release of these stress hormones from the organs works great during acute stress, but produces negative effects when in chronic stress. After the fight or flight stage, your body will try to get back to a homeostasis stage to bring your whole system back to normal. However, if there's a prolonged stressor, your body will become alarmed and move from homeostasis to the resistance stage.

The resistance stage is where the stressors prolong and your body will keep on producing hormones, which is how your body responds for long term protection. This is where the stress hormones becomes damaging to your body. You may feel regular tiredness, a lack of enthusiasm, regular infections, and a lower sex drive. This phase might continue for several months or even years.

This is why constant breaks with breathing, stretches, and taking less than a minute out of every hour to become mindful play an important role in our daily life. The ten strategies following this chapter will help you achieve this goal.

Digestive System

When you are under stress, your central nerves system shuts down blood circulation to your digestive system to prepare your arms, legs, and head for quick thinking, to fight or to flee. This response is good when it's during fight or flight, but when there are prolonged stressors or stress becomes chronic, it becomes harmful and may contribute to, or cause, stomach ulcers, irritable bowel syndrome (IBS), and food allergies.

In an article posted by Dr. Mercola, "How Stress Wrecks Havoc on Your Gut -- And What to Do About it" which cites Harvard reviews, Mercola explains how stress can   cause stomach disorders and a damage gut can contribute to diseases and conditions such as multiple sclerosis, rheumatoid arthritis, lupus, Crohn's disease, chronic skin conditions, urinary conditions, and degenerative conditions[6].

From the same article, "The Harvard HealthBeat has compiled a useful list of physical, behavioral and emotional symptoms of stress. We're all exposed to stress virtually every day, but these signs signal that stress may have become overwhelming in your life, and could be increasing your risk of related health problems."

Here are some of the symptoms shared from Harvard HealthBeat:

Physical Symptoms:

- Stiff muscles, especially in the neck and shoulders
- Headaches
- Sleep problems
- Recent loss of interest in sex
- Weight loss or gain

Behavioral Symptoms:

- Procrastination
- Grinding teeth
- Difficulty completing work assignment
- Taking up smoking, or smoking more than usual

Emotional Symptoms:

- Overwhelming sense of tension or pressure
- Trouble relaxing
- Depression

---

6 "How Does Stress Wreak Havoc on Your Gut? - Mercola." 2012.
<http://articles.mercola.com/sites/articles/archive/2012/04/09/chronic-stress-gut-effects.aspx>

- Having a hard time remembering thing
- Indecisiveness

How Can You Do To Reduce Stress And Improve Your Gut Health?

- Exercise isn't restrained to just going to the gym, a simple half hour walk around the neighborhood, or if it is cool, drive to the mall and window shop for half hour
- Get a massage - ask to include a colon massage in your session
- Yoga
- Deep breathing
- Avoid sugar or anything that has fructose
- **Incorporate** any of the *10 strategies from the following chapters* to prevent or lessen your stress

Nervous System

Our nervous system is divided into two parts: the somatic system (which takes care of the decision making, consciousness, and intelligence) and the autonomic nervous system (also known as ANS, which keeps your heart beating, controls the acidity of your stomach, and amount of sugar in your blood) does the functions beyond your consciousness. The autonomic system is also divided into sympathetic nervous system SNS and parasympathetic nervous system PNS.

The sympathetic nervous system helps you to respond to stressors, prepare your body to respond to fight or flight. The parasympathetic nervous system does the opposite of the sympathetic system by calming down the heart rate, regulates the glands by producing saliva or tears, and stimulates secretions in the digestive system[7].

---

[7] "How stress affects your body - Ben Benjamin." 2007.
<http://www.benbenjamin.com/pdfs/Issue6.pdf>

The sympathetic nervous system is designed to take care of stress, and the parasympathetic nervous system is designed to calm things down, like the Chinese Yin and Yang (Yin representing the bright or positive side of things and Yang the dark or negative side.)

The autonomic system controls the heart, the blood vessels, temperature control like blushing, breathing, the digestive system, filling the bladder, but not emptying it, and most aspects of the reproductive system. How your autonomic system runs depends on the amount of stress you are experiencing in your life.

Some symptoms that you might want to note[8]:

- Your voice starts to croak when confronted by your boss.
- When you sweat more than usual.
- Blush readily.
- Heart races readily.
- Bladder control problems.

17 Reasons to AVOID STRESS

I want to share some information from an infographic by Fawne Hansen at The Adrenal Fatigue Solution.[9]

1. ***Headaches*** - Increasing number of headaches in a month is high stress related.

2. ***Hair Loss*** - Women with high stress experience hair loss and hair thinning.

3. ***Memory*** - Chronic stress has been linked to damaging neurotransmitters, which weakens memory.

---

8   "How Does Stress Affects Your Nervous System | Medical Site." 2013. <http://www.medicalsite.info/stress/how-does-stress-affects-your-nervous-system/>
9   "17 Reasons To Avoid Stress: An Infographic." 2014. <http://adrenalfatiguesolution.com/17-reasons-to-avoid-stress/>

4. ***Acne / Psoriasis*** - Acne increases in students with high stress, especially during exams.

5. ***Insomnia*** - Poor psychosocial working environment increase the risk of developing insomnia.

6. ***Heart Attacks*** - 23% employee with stressful jobs are likely to have heart attack.

7. ***Worsens Asthma*** - Chronic stress doubles the risk of asthma.

8. ***Sugar Craving*** - High levels of stress hormones lead to craving sweet food.

9. ***Digestion*** - The constant turning on and off of chronic stress interrupts the digestive system.

10. ***Belly Fat*** - High levels of cortisol from stress causes excess fat in the abdominal region.

11. ***Back Pain*** - High levels of cortisol from stress has been associated with chronic back pain.

12. ***Sex Drive*** - High levels of cortisol from stress affect sexual functions.

13. ***Blood Pressure*** - Stress increase blood pressure that may create heart problems.

14. ***Adrenal Fatigue*** - Chronic stress can weaken hormone production that can cause fatigue and low immunity.

15. ***Blood Sugar*** - 45% of men with permanent stress may develop Type II diabetes from hormones elevated by stress.

16. ***Aging*** - Chronic stress affect telomere length, which indicate premature aging.

17. ***Immune System*** - Constant prolonged stress weaken immune system.

Your stress stops here! You can use any of the strategies in this book at to help relieve stress. With the help of the mindfulness bell, or any reminder app, take a break to use these strategies every hour when you are at work or when you are in a stressful situation.

Email your receipt from Amazon to the email below now. Download *Your Stress Stops Here! Journal* so that you can keep a good record and see your progress.

Email your Amazon Receipt To:
join-stress@0s4.com

CHAPTER 3

Push And Rub Strategy (Base Of Skull)

---

*"Life is not about how fast you run,
or how high you climb, but how well you bounce."*

- Unknown

Have you ever experienced a combination of neck pain and tightness of the muscles at the base of the skull? Do you remember what caused the pain? What do you think are the major causes of the pain?

The pain could be caused by:

- Spending too much time on the computer.
- Spending too much time on the phone.
- Probably from an accident.
- Posture - how you hold your head.

Most of the pain behind the *skull and on your neck* comes from spending too much time on the computer. Staring into the computer, reading books, watching television for a long period of time with an improper position, and cradling the phone on your neck can easily strain the area. Your posture also plays a big role in it. (See Chapter 4 - Row Backwards Strategy) One quick tip! Whenever you have a pain, always try to trace it back to the activities, or maybe sometimes what you eat, before the pain happened.

The IT Guy

John works in the IT department of a top shoe designer corporate office in New York. John works out five times a week and even joined the Israel boot camp twice a week (a health program offered by the company). The company had just added a new wing, and he has to do the ordering of the hardware, setting up of the hardware, and have the system up and going. The wiring and cables were put in by a cable installation company and finished as promised. The project was going pretty smooth for the first few weeks until the hardware arrived at the office. Only ten out of fifteen sets of the hardware came. He has to call and follow up with the company he ordered from while trying to start setting up with what he had. He was relieved when the rest of the order arrived, but came to find out that a few of the parts were missing. So, he had to get back to the phone to call the company again. He began to stress out about the missing parts, and on top of that, the deadline coming up soon made it worse. The missing parts came two days later. Just as he thought everything was on track, there was a system problem on a different system with another department. He had to stop what he was doing and move to the problem in the other department.

He *spent a lot of time* in front of the computer, sometimes *working until 11:30* at night trying to find a solution to the problem. He began to work out less because of all the time demanded by his work. He had just become a first time father two months prior to the new project. He felt that his *stress level was increasing* and he *hadn't had enough sleep* since the arrival of his baby boy.

When John was experiencing *all these stresses*, I was the in-house therapist at that company twice a week (another health program offered by that company). He came to me one Thursday with *pain on the base of the skull and some neck pain*. I asked him how the pain came about, and he told me how it started. He told me how many times he works out, how he had to work on the new project, how he had to face one problem after another, and how he has to work the night shift to take care of the baby. The pressure of meeting the deadline and fixing the system problem has *caused the pain for him*. I continued to ask him if he had done something physically that might have caused the pain. He remembered something *felt funny on his neck* while he was lifting. He also remembered that he has to pat his son to sleep while carrying him on the shoulder.

His story reminded me of what I did while I was working in corporate America. I remembered having to spend many hours keying in payments into the system, carrying boxes of invoices to the computer for printing, and the pressure from the month end billing and deadlines for reports to be generated.

I began to feel his shoulder and neck for tight spots (sometime call knots, these are the areas where there's a lot tension in a muscle or a group of muscles). I was able to find the spots easily because of the clues I got from his complaints and answers from me asking him what he thought happened. I made him to think on anything else he recently did right before the pain. I worked on him for 20 minutes, and he felt much better. I also asked him to follow up by doing the push and rub strategy himself two times a day or when he feels the tension reoccuring.

Push And Rub Base Of Skull Strategy:

Now that you know what the causes the pain underneath your skull and neck, it's time to figure out how to relieve the pain by yourself. Ok! Let me show you a quick and simple technique that I use to release this pain.

Step 1

You need to use the side of your hand, the soft cushiony part right under your pinky (I am going to call it the side of the hand from now on). Start with the side that's most uncomfortable.

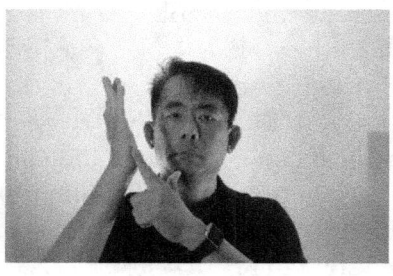

- Place your hand 45° under the base of the skull.
- Push the side of your hand into the base of the skull.
- Do the same all along the neck.
- Push the muscle with the corner of your palm and jiggle (this action will help loosen the muscle and also get deeper into the muscle.

Step 2

- Use the side of your hand and rub into the base of the skull. Do it as if you are sawing the area with your side of the hand, start slowly and increase the speed until you feel warm on your base of the skull and the side of the neck.
- You can combine the pushing and the rubbing action.

Step 3

Once it's all nice and warm, you can start working on the other side.

- Place your hand 45° under the base of the skull.
- Push the side of your hand into the base of the skull.
- Do the same all along the neck.
- Push the muscle with the corner of your palm and

jiggle. This action will help loosen the muscle and also to get deeper into the muscle.

Step 4

- Use the side of your hand and rub into the base of the skull. Do it as if you are sawing the area with your side of the hand. Start slowly and increase the speed until you feel warm on your base of the skull and the side of the neck.
- You can combine the pushing and the rubbing action.

Step 5 TO END

- Use both the palm of your hands.
- Move them up and down as if you are swiping your neck to the base of the skull with your palm instead of your finger.
- Do this five times, but do it really fast for the last two (until you feel like your neck is fully heated).

Why do you want to rub it fast?

When you rub it fast, you bring blood and circulation to the area; you'll actually feel the heat. After that quick movement, you'll feel the whole neck heated up, which is a good thing. That means you actually brought circulation to the area and the blood is flowing. You'll feel the relief right away. When there is circulation, there is oxygen; when there's oxygen, there's no pain. Where there's no pain, there's no stress!

Your stress stops here! You can use any of the strategies in this book at to help relieve stress. With the help of the mindfulness bell, or any reminder app, take a break to use these strategies every hour when you are at work or when you are in a stressful situation.

Bonus: Push And Rub Strategy (Video)

Go ahead and **email your receipt from Amazon to the email below now** to see how it's done. Download *Your Stress Stops Here! Journal* so that you can keep a good record and see your progress.

Email your Amazon Receipt To:
join-stress@0s4.com

CHAPTER 4

Row Backward Strategy (Neck & Back)

"Stress is the trash of modern life — we all generate it,
but if you don't dispose of it properly,
it will pile up and overtake your life."

- Danzae Pace

Do not hunch when sitting! Sit up straight! Push your chest forward! Straighten your shoulders! Stop slouching or hunching! Sit all the way back! Make sure you have good posture, otherwise the girls will not like you! Have you heard these statements or commands from your parents or teachers when you were younger? You might have heard at least one or more of those, or something similar to these, in your lifetime. These were told to us and should be part of our life or should be known as common sense, but sometimes common sense might not be so common after all. You probably can relate to this. You   know when your parents reminded you to do something that you knew you should do, but you never do it anyways.

My parents always reminded me to sit up straight, but they never actually showed me how to do it right. It took me a long time to figure it out. It wasn't until I learned it in massage school when I understand the muscles involved and the mechanics of holding a good posture. I also learned that every muscle, movement, and organ in our body works together as a whole. I always say, "If you mess up your ankle, you will mess up your knee. If you mess up your knee, you will your mess up your lower back. If you mess up your lower back, you will mess up your upper back and shoulder. If you mess up your upper back and shoulder, you will mess up your neck. If you mess up your neck, you will mess up your head."

We tend to find the easy way out by sitting wrong and later on wonder why we were not feeling well or feeling pain. Yes! I said not feeling well or pain. Your body will slowly adapt to this changes when it is repeated daily, intentionally or unintentionally, and eventually cause pain or might even bring toll to your body.

Let's take a look what happens to your body when you are slouching, hunching over, or not sitting properly. Your neck is forward, shoulders curve towards the front, and your lower back is pushed backwards. What could cause you to be in this position at work, at home, or even when you are driving? Can you guess? You are right! Working intensely in front of or staring at the computer and also grinding or crunching your teeth (we'll talk about this later in the facial tension section), watching movies on your phone, iPad, or tablet, and stressing out by holding tightly to the steering wheel during traffic jams, typing and cradling the phone between your shoulder, and last but not least, sitting too long without taking any breaks. This was one of the biggest factors that cause all the pains that I had when I was working in corporate America.)

Neck pain, shoulder pain, and lower back pain are caused by bad posture alone. These will cause your chest muscles to tighten up, your back muscles to loosen or stretch out, and your lower back muscles to tense. Do you know that slouching may

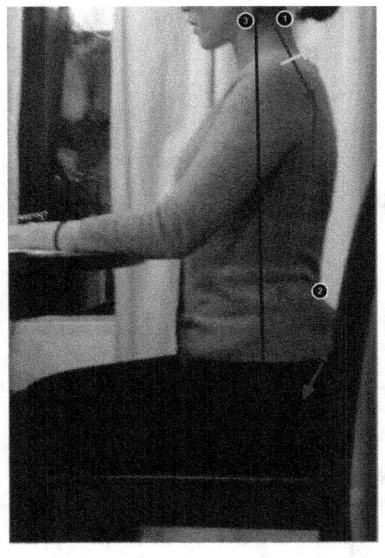

also cause digestive distress? Try slouching and then try sitting up straight the next time you go to the bathroom, you will notice the difference. You will go faster and easier when you sit up straight compared to slouching because when you are slouching, you put pressure on to your intestines; this creates blockage instead of direct flow.

We will first look into how you should sit and then look at the strategy you can use to solve this situation.

I've learned that many people sit on their tailbone, which is the tiny piece of bone right under their sacrum (that's the piece of bone that looks like a triangle that holds their pelvis together). The correct way is to sit with your sit bone (this is the bone that's on the cheek of your butt).

A good or healthy back should have three curves:

- curve at the neck
- curve at the upper back (area below the shoulder before the lower back)
- curve at the lumbar (lower back area)

When you sit, your shoulders should be level on both sides (green line), upper back should be curved (chest forward) and lower back should be curved (#2) The red line (#1) shows how the spine should be. The blue line (#3) gives you an idea of how your head, shoulders, and sit bones should align.

Your arms should be level with the desk (you can adjust the height of the chair). Your feet should be completely flat on the floor. You can use a foot rest if your feet don't touch the floor. It is important to have your feet supported because if they are not supported, it may cause tension to the back of your feet. It will also cause you to slip off the chair. Your computer screen should be at your eye level (you can use a box or a monitor stand to elevate it) and should be an arm's length or 18-24 inches away.

If you haven't tried yet, you can try this posture right now and feel the difference immediately. Sitting up straight this way actually makes you more confident. It also allows you to breathe better.

Importance Of Taking A Break

Take a break after spending 55 minutes to an hour staring at the computer. Stand up and take a water break (make sure you drink at least 6 to 8 cups of clean filtered water to clean your internal system) or take a pee break. I always tell my clients to do so because it's only fair for them to take a water break or a pee break when their colleagues get to go outside for a cigarette smoke break. During these breaks, you can refocus by doing head to knees and row backward strategies, which you will learn about in this chapter. I use a mindfulness bell to remind me when I'm using my computer. I also use the activity app on my Apple watch. If you have an Apple watch, you can use the activity app. This will remind you to stand up every hour on the hour. You need to get a reminder app on your phone or computer. Here are some of the ones I recommend:

- The Fungie Mindfullness Bell - http://fungie.info/bell/#

- Mindful Clock - http://www.mindfulnessdc.org/mindfulclock.html

- Insight Timer - https://www.InsightTimer.com. It's free and works for iphones and androids.

- Lotus Bud Mindfulness Bell - https://itunes.apple.com/us/app/lotus-bud-

mindfulness-bell/id502329366?mt=8
It's free and works for iphones.

- Re.minder -
https://itunes.apple.com/us/app/re.minder/
id395529341?mt=8.
It's free and works for iphones/

Row Backwards Strategy: (Neck & Back Head To Knee)

Step 1

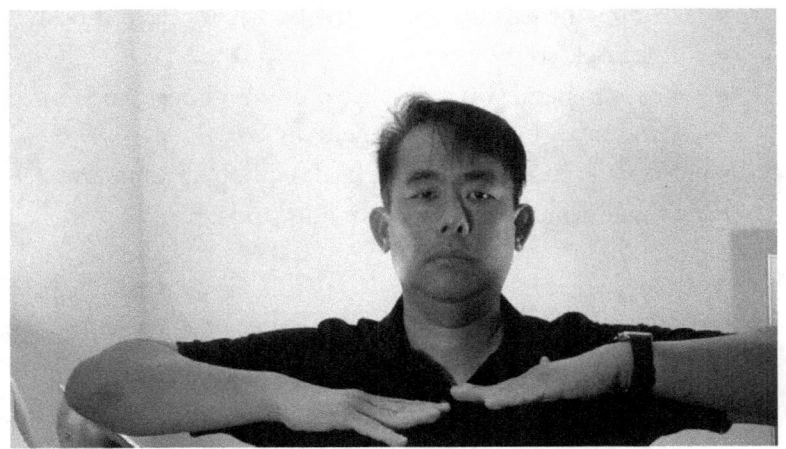

- Put your arms up straight like you are reaching out in front of you, parallel to your shoulders.

- Bring your hands in towards your chest (fingers pointing towards each other).

- Breathe in, slowly move your shoulders backwards, and at the same time, slowly move your forearm diagonally up until your hands are in a surrender position.

- Stop once you feel like your shoulder blades are touching each other or your shoulder blade area tightens up. **Note - DO NOT** *overdo it! Just move until it tightens and NOT until it hurts.***

- Breathe out slowly, bring your hands to the sides of your body, and relax.

Take a couple of deep breaths and rest for 30 seconds.

Step 2

Head to knees

- Stand up, legs parallel and a foot apart from each other.
- Bring your hands towards the back of your mid-body.
- Interlock your fingers.
- Begin to bend your head towards your knees, and at the same time, point your fingers upwards.
- You will hear your upper back getting an adjustment.
- Slowly come back to the standing position.

The row backwards strategy helps release the chest muscles from tightening up, your back muscles go back to normal and tension on your lower back is gone.

Your stress stops here! You can use any of the strategies in this book at to help relieve stress. With the help of the mindfulness bell, or any reminder app, take a break to use these strategies every hour when you are at work or when you are in a stressful situation.

Bonus: Row Backward Strategy (Video)

Go ahead and **email your receipt from Amazon to the email below now** to see how it's done. Download *Your Stress Stops Here! Journal* so that you can keep a good record and see your progress.

Email your Amazon Receipt To:
join-stress@0s4.com

CHAPTER 5

Yawn Away Strategy (Stress)

"Working hard for something we don't care about is called stress. Working hard for something we love is called passion."

- Simon Sinek

A Typical Workday

April is a director of technical design in the fashion industry in New York City.   She is in charge of five divisions, or brands, in the company. She wakes up at 5:45 A.M. and leaves the house by 7:00 A.M. She arrives at work before 8:00 A.M., turns on the computer, and has breakfast while answering her work emails. Knowing her, she would answer her emails in the subway if there's internet or a WiFi connection. She answers her emails until 9:00 AM and attends the first fitting until 11 A.M. or noon, goes back to her desk, and continues to read her emails. She eats lunch at her desk while answering more emails until her next fitting at 2 P.M. until 4 P.M. Then she goes back to her desk to *catch up* with her daily tasks.

Once her department received the sample from the vendors, they have to count how many samples received and estimate how much *time they need* then to book the fit model ahead of time. Before the fitting, all samples are *checked, prepared, and measured,* then she goes to the fitting with production, merchandising, design, and her own team. They'll put the garment on the fit model, *evaluate for any fix issues,* and design will *give their input.* Then her team will *note all the corrections* (if the arm hole fits, sleeve is too long or shoulder seam is falling to the back) and move to the next sample.

After fitting, she has to go back to her desk and starts to *enter all (pictures, notes, changes) fit comments* into an *old system* which has *a lot of problems,* but it's the only system they have. She has to think about the spec measurements and *enter fit comments* to address the fit issues. She checks the construction of the garment to make sure the label is positioned correctly. At the end of the day, she posts an email notification of all the completed fit comments to their overseas vendors

Each season starts with the merchandise team choosing the assortment for the deliveries. Then the team *fits the samples* and *adjusts the fit* until it's ready for manufacturing. Her team is *responsible for assisting* design to develop line, review samples, fit samples, and *correct* them for production. April is *in charge of five divisions,* which means she has to go through the entire garment lifecycle with all five divisions, five seasons a year; that's 25 times per season *(which is a lot of work)*! The stages of the *seasons always overlap.* For example, when they are ready for fall production stage of fall season, it's also first fit for winter season and development stage for spring season.

Every week, April has to *plan, schedule, and divide* the workload and make sure the fit comments are sent out on time. She checks her email to make sure all the urgent issues are addressed, looks at her calendar to make sure the whole week's event are covered, schedules fittings and   attends meetings.

Everyday an unplanned event comes up, and she has to deal with it and get the work done.

You can see how April could be *overwhelmed and buried* with all the work that's put upon her. She comes to me every week for stress relief, and I showed her the next strategy. Every week, I would remind her to work on herself with the strategies that I am showing you in this book.

Do you know that *yawning helps release your stress?* I thought it was weird when I first heard about this. I said to myself, "What does yawning have to do with stress relief?" but I accepted it with an open mind. I like trying out new things, especially the weird stuff. Yawning helps stimulate alertness and concentration, increases memory recall, increases productivity, lowers stress, and relaxes the body.

Yawning is being use by managers, CEOs, core leaders of multi-million dollars companies who can't afford to have any physical or mental stress in their life. They pay a lot of money to learn this strategy, plus five others according to Mark Waldman, the co-author of *How God Changes Your Brain*[10].

I use it on myself and it works, although my wife asks me why am I always yawning. I also used this strategy to help me write this book (imagine me yawning every 55 minutes!). I use this strategy more than the next strategy which is the rub and release strategy for facial tension because it is convenient and doesn't require much.

You may be thinking, "I can't yawn, I'm not tired, or how do I yawn on demand?" Well, if managers, CEO, and core leaders are using this strategy, why don't you give it a try? All you have to do is fake the first few yawns, and then you will automatically start yawning by the fifth or sixth. Pay attention and be aware of how much your stress level falls.

The yawn away strategy is great to use whenever you have anger, anxiety, or stress:

---

[10] "god_newberg - baillement.com." 2011.
<http://www.baillement.com/dossier/god_newberg.html>

- Close your eyes.

- Breathe in and fake the first few (yawn 10 times). With each yawn, bring in a quality of mindfulness and get into the present moment. By the fifth or sixth yawn, you will feel the amount of stress lessen.

- Continue to 10 or more.

Although we were told that yawning in front of someone may seem impolite, the effects of yawning can mean a lot to those who are stressed. It can stimulate alertness, concentration, increase memory, increase productivity, lower stress, and relax the body. So yawn away when you feel stress!

Your stress stops here! You can use any of the strategies in this book at to help relieve stress. With the help of the mindfulness bell, or any reminder app, take a break to use these strategies every hour when you are at work or when you are in a stressful situation.

Bonus: Yawn Away Strategy (Video)

Go ahead and **email your receipt from Amazon to the email below now** to see how it's done. Download *Your Stress Stops Here! Journal* so that you can keep a good record and see your progress.

Email your Amazon Receipt To:
join-stress@0s4.com

CHAPTER 6

Rub and Release
Strategy (Eyes & Face)

---

*"Sometimes the most important thing in a whole day
is the rest we take between two deep breaths."*

- *Etty Hillesum*

Computer Vision Syndrome / Digital Eyestrain

With the quick advancement of technology and gadgets, most people spend a lot of time *in front of their computer screen*, both at work and at home, and more so with the use of smartphones and tablets (I'm guilty of this!). Do you know that *staring at* the computer screen, smartphone, and tablet for a period of time may *strain your eyes* and will worsen your existing condition? The American Optometric Association calls it computer vision syndrome, or digital eyestrain, for *extended use* of computers and other digital devices.[11]

---

[11] "Eyestrain Causes - Mayo Clinic." 2014. <http://www.mayoclinic.org/diseases-conditions/eyestrain/basics/causes/con-20032649>

The causes of the *eyestrain,* besides spending extended hours on computers and digital devices, are: reading *without* taking a break, not using *proper lighting,* and *being stressed* or fatigued. *Sore neck, sore shoulder* or *sore back,* and *tired eyes* are some of the *symptoms of eyestrain.*

According to Dr. Blakeney, an optometric adviser to the College of Optometrists, the position of the computer screen should be in front of you. The eyes are positioned so that they *look straight ahead and slightly down.* The top of the screen should be *in line with your eye level.* The screen should be placed approximately *18-30 inches away from you.* Use an *anti-glare screen,* or if you wear glasses, make sure you get *anti-glare lenses* or simply place blinds over nearby windows. *Tilting your computer screen* 10-15 degrees slightly backwards helps with the glare from ceiling lighting[12].

Staring at the computer screen for an extended amount of time will *dry up your eyes* because when you stare and concentrate, you tend to blink less or sometimes, we do not to blink at all. Your body generates its own medicine. You can moisten your eyes by *simply blinking* your eyes; the eyes will secrete natural fluid to moist them. You may also *use eye drops.* Combine blinking or using eye drops with the rub and release strategy; you'll feel great and refreshed.

Facial Expression

Imagine being *stressed by holding onto your steering wheel really tightly* during rush hour and having to *concentrate* more on the road when there are traffic jams, the doctor *told you* that someone you love needs a surgery to save his or her live, you are *working intensely* in front of, or *staring at, the computer* and also *grinding or crunching your teeth,* someone just *said no* to something you really wanted, you have a *deadline to meet* (how I'm feeling right now!).

I started thinking about and actually working on this book

---

12 "does looking at a computer damage your eyes - news medical." 2012. <http://www.news-medical.net/health/Does-looking-at-a-computer-damage-your-eyes.aspx>

about a month ago. I had an idea about what I wanted for the book in my head, but it's a little different when it comes to actually writing it. I *spend at least five hours* a day in front of the computer screen, plus *research* on the iPad (hint hint, digital eye strain). I pay attention to *my posture* when I'm writing and doing my research, making sure *my back is properly curved, my head, shoulders, and sit bone are aligned,* my computer screen is 10- 15 degrees tilted backwards, and it's 18 to 30 inches away, or an arm's length away, from me at my eye level. I change my writing venues from the living room to the dining room, to my office, to my daughter's room, and my local library just to *prevent stress* and writing blocks.

Although I took precautions with my posture, the ergonomics, my change of venue, I still felt stress. I personally felt stress, yes. I noticed that *when I'm stressed,* I *tend to crunch my teeth.* When you are stressed, *do you do the "hmm"* and you don't realize that you are *tightening up your teeth and your jaw?* I felt the same when I tend to t*hink a little harder* when doing my regular work, when I go grocery shopping, *stuck in traffic, getting ready for dinner,* or even shopping at the mall, except for Apple store!

What happens to your *facial muscles when you are stressed? Your eyes get strained,* your *temple muscles tighten, your cheek muscles tighten as you crunch your teeth, which leads to tightening your jaw muscle.* In short, you get tired or strained eyes and a face with tightened muscles. I found the best and easiest way to *prevent all* this is to smile no matter what. *Smile* when you are happy, and smile when you are stressed.

I use the rub and release strategy on the president of the shoe company (the same company with John the IT guy in Chapter Three). He was always *moving* from one meeting to another and *highly stressed.* In the beginning, he would spend some time on the phone when he came into the treatment room. After a few months, he realized the i*mportance of being relaxed and let go;* he would just come into the room and put on his music and relax. I would always end with the rub and release strategy on him, and he always walked out of the treatment room with a smile.

First, I'm going to show you how to use the rub and release strategy on your eyes.

What do you do if you still strain your eyes, in spite of what was suggested above (placing your computer screen 18 to 30 inches away at eye level and take frequent breaks)? This is where the rub and release strategy comes into play.

Before you start, I want you to take a look at the mirror and just take a minute to look at your face. Keep that image somewhere in your brain or maybe take a selfie so that you can compare the before and after look.

Rub and release strategy for the **eyes***:*

Step 1

- Put both your hands together.
- Fingers interlocking with each other.
- Palms facing each other.
- Rub them together until you feel warm/heat on your palms.
- Close your eyes and place your warm palms on each eye until you feel the heat diminish.

Do this two times.

Step 2

- Put both your hands together.
- Fingers interlocking with each other.
- Palms facing each other.
- Rub them together until you feel warm/heat on your palms.
- Close your eyes, **BUT this time** wipe your eyes with your warm palms (like the windshield wiper of your car) one on each eye slowly from the ridge of your nose and outward five times or until the heat diminishes.

Do this two times.

Step 3 to finish up

Repeat Step 1, *BUT only once.*

Next, I'm going to go through the rub and release strategy for the rest of the face.

Once your facial muscles tighten, your jaw muscles will also tighten up due to the crunching of your teeth.

*Rub and release strategy for the **face**:*

Step 1

- Rub your hand together until you feel the heat.
- Wipe your face from the ridge of your nose outwards five times (like you are dividing it into two).

Do this two times.

Step 2

- Use the pad of your finger tip.
- Gently rub your forehead with both hands; start with the middle of your forehead and do a circular motion moving outwards on both sides.

Step 3

- Use the pad of your finger tip.
- Gently rub your cheek from under your eye with a circular motion moving outwards.
- Do the same for the lower cheek starting from the area parallel to your nose and outwards.
- Finally, rub your chin from the middle of your lips with a circular motion moving outwards.

As you are using this strategy, I want you to notice how your muscles begin to loosen up; enjoy that feeling.

Step 4

- Draw a line from the middle of your nose; move your hand towards your earlobe to find the spot where your jaw bone connects to your skull (you can locate it by dropping your jaw).
- Rub the spot with circular movement and drop your jaw as you rub it.

Repeat this until you feel relief on the jaw.
You can add in the 360 slow motion while doing the above steps. The 360 slow motion will help release tension in the neck and shoulders.

Step 5

- Tap on your face all over slowly, start from the forehead.
- Tap slowly around your eye.
- Tap on your cheek and move on to the chin.

Step 6

- Rub your hands together until you feel the heat.
- Cover your face with your hands until the heat fades off.

Congratulations! You have just completed the rub and release strategy on yourself...in the spa world, this means you just gave yourself a facial massage! Go check out your face and see the difference. Take another selfie and compare them. Share it on our private Facebook page!

Your stress stops here! You can use any of the strategies in this book at to help relieve stress. With the help of the mindfulness bell, or any reminder app, take a break to use these strategies every hour when you are at work or when you are in a stressful situation.

> ### *Bonus: Rub and Release Strategy (Video)*
>
> **Go ahead** and **email your receipt from Amazon to the email below now** to see how it's done. Download *Your Stress Stops Here! Journal* so that you can keep a good record and see your progress.
>
> *Email your Amazon Receipt To:*
> *join-stress@0s4.com*

CHAPTER 7

Press And Move Strategy (Shoulder, Shoulder Blade)

"Unnatural work produces too much stress."

- Bhagavad Gita

Do you or you know someone *having problems with their shoulders*? Have you been *sleeping on one side*? Did you wake up with a *pain in the shoulder*? Does your shoulder bother you? Did you *hurt your shoulder* shoveling too much snow?

When I woke up this morning, I felt the pain in my shoulder by the joint and to the shoulder blade. Why? I think it's because lately I haven't been sleeping with the proper pillow positioning. This happens once in awhile, and what do you normally do? What should you do?

Do you *sleep on your side*? Do you know that when you sleep on the side, most of your weight is shifted to the side you sleep on? For example, when you sleep on your left side, most of your body weight, in fact all of your body weight, is on to the left side. Do you know that it will cause pain if you do not *sleep properly*? You need to *prop your pillows* so that you will not put *weight on only one shoulder*.

Rebuilding The House

Ben was in the process of rebuilding his house. He tore down the interior of the house because it was old and was weirdly built. The space wasn't properly utilized and everything felt close and tight. He decided to save some money by doing most of the work himself. During this time, he had to *put up with his relative* and ended up *sleeping on the couch*. The couch is not an ideal place to sleep because it brings *more aches and pain* than a good night rest. The *improper sleeping condition* and the reconstruction of the house created stress in his shoulder and shoulder blade. I found out that he was *sleeping on his side* all this time. He had put his whole body weight on to his left side, and his left shoulder and shoulder blade was feeling the effect from his sleeping position.

Old Injury

My family and I were invited by my wife's family friend (we are going to call her "Yuki" because she's from Japan) to vacation in Hawaii for Christmas. Yuki owns a construction company in Japan. Her company does major construction and repairs for the Japanese government. Yuki works very hard and sometimes, when there's not enough help, she'll chip in to help. There was one time when she helped *carry ten fifty pounds cement bags* at a construction site when she was a worker short. We were so happy to see her and her family. While catching up, she told us how she has to finish up her projects before her vacation and the end of the year, and was so ready to play golf.

The flight from Japan to Hawaii wasn't that long, but she felt a little stress in the neck and back area. I took a look by feeling her neck, shoulder, and upper back, and I found tightness on the *shoulder and the shoulder blades*. As usual, I started to do some investigative work, like I do with all of my clients, by asking her what she thought was the cause of it, if she had *an accident or hurt the area* before and what was she doing before *the pain occurred.* I came to find out about her *hurting herself* while carrying the bags of cement two years ago. Additionally, one of her sisters, who was *very dear to her, passed away* six months prior to her vacation. She didn't get *any therapy for the injury* because she thought it *wasn't a major injury* and let it subside.

My advice to her and you (if you had an accident or hurt yourself) is *have it checked out and get therapy.* WHY? If you *do not take care* of it in the early stage, it will *come back to haunt you* later in life. When it does come to haunt you, you might not even remember what happened. *Any injury not taken care of right away* will end up with *scar tissue, and you will feel pain,* even with a little stress to the area.

Let me show you the press and move strategy to release the pain on the joint area and also the shoulder blade.

Press And Move Strategy

First: *To loosen up the **shoulder***

Step 1

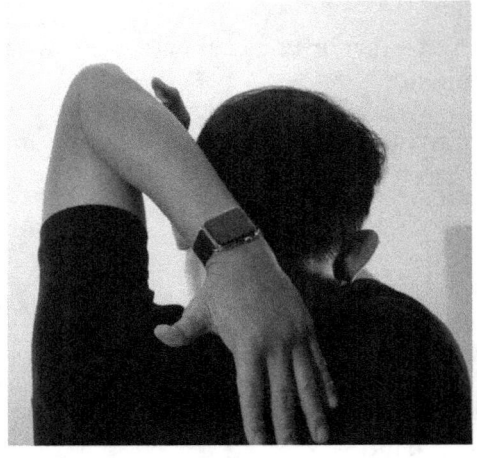

- Lift your hand up, bend your elbow, and push your elbow down with your other hand.

Release and Repeat three times.

Step 2

Switch hands

- Lift your hand up, bend your elbow, and push your elbow down with your other hand.

Release and Repeat three times.

Second: *to loosen up the* **shoulder blades**

- Put your arms out sideways perpendicular to the shoulders (imagine you are doing the airplane when you were younger).
- Start moving your hands slowly like you are drawing a small circle.
- Start moving your hands slowly like you are drawing a medium circle.
- Start moving your hands slowly like you are drawing a large circle.
- Start moving your hands slowly like you are drawing an extra large circle.

Step 3

Third:

- Find the tight spot.
- Put a little pressure on it with your finger pads of your opposite hand.

- Lift the elbow of the hand where the tight spot is.

- Move that hand forward and backwards as if you are rowing a boat.

Work on it until you feel the spot loosen (meaning the tight spot becomes soft and there is no pain).
When done, move to the next spot.

Repeat Step 3

Keep repeating Step 3 until you feel the whole area is nice and soft.
You now know what to do when you have tense shoulder or shoulder blade. You can use this strategy as soon as you feel the tension coming. The sooner you address it, the sooner you prevent the stress from affecting you!

Your stress stops here! You can use any of the strategies in this book at to help relieve stress. With the help of the mindfulness bell, or any reminder app, take a break to use these strategies every hour when you are at work or when you are in a stressful situation.

Bonus: Press And Move Strategy (Video)

Go ahead and **email your receipt from Amazon to the email below now** to see how it's done. Download **Your Stress Stops Here! Journal** so that you can keep a good record and see your progress.

Email your Amazon Receipt To:
join-stress@0s4.com

CHAPTER 8

Run For Your Life
Strategy (Stress)

---

*"At times of great stress, it is especially necessary
to achieve a complete freeing of the muscles."*

- - *Konstantin Stanislavsky*

D o you work at a place where as soon as you step into your
workplace, you start working and don't stop until it's time
to go home? Do you have a job that whenever you stress, you
need to snap out of it, *refocus* and then get back to work? In most
companies, you get *more responsibility and a heavier workload* when
you are given a promotion. I remembered that my responsibility
and workload tripled as soon as I was promoted from a
freelancer to a supervisor while working in corporate America. I
had to finish my work and on top of that, I had to make sure
my team under my supervision finished or had their work up to
date.

I had to put in the *overtime* if any of them weren't   current with their task. It was *always stressful* when it came to the end of the month or when someone was sick in my department. Guess what? We always have that one person who always sick. It was a unionized company, as long as you bring a doctor's note, upper management cannot do anything about it. The *stress increased* when upper management wanted special reports when sales weren't good.

Billy

Ms. Anderson is a fourth grade teacher in a public school in suburban New Jersey. She has 22 students in her class. Like most teachers, she has a mix of some good, some talkative, some active, some quiet, and one ADHD kid. Billy has a history of getting whatever he wants at home. When Billy was in second grade, he refused to do his lesson in class. Billy pushed his books off his desk, hid under his desk, and refused to get up from under his desk. The principal had to call in the town's police to make him come out from under the desk.

That was two years ago; Billy now gets a teacher's assistant sitting next to him helping him with his school work. He has been fine from the beginning of the school year, but acted up last week. This time Billy didn't want to do his class work in class and wanted to do it at home instead, so he had a tantrum. He *slapped* Ms. Anderson and kicked the teacher's assistant. Ms. Anderson has to call in the dean to handle the situation. Ms. Anderson had to spend a third of the class time catering to Billy. She felt that that was unfair for the rest of the students. We can see *how stressful* it can be for Ms. Anderson and her assistant in situations like this.

Chef Wong

Chef Wong (a friend of mine when I was working at the restaurant) was a chef for at *busy* restaurant in midtown Manhattan. He and his team go in the restaurant at 10 A.M. to prepare the food for the menu of the day. He has to make sure his cold (salad and cold sandwiches) station and hot (burgers and hot food) station teams have their prep work done by 11:30 A.M. (when the restaurant opens for lunch). Chef Wong goes into work and *does not stop* until 2:30 P.M. every time he works. His duties included ordering the meats, vegetables, *foreseeing all prep work*, figuring out the specials for each day, experimenting new dishes, making sure the dishes are well presented, and also his team's schedules.

In the midst of all the craziness, Chef Wong and his team would take some *time to de-stress* by doing jumping jacks ten times really quickly. He told me that that's what he did as a stretch in school when he was in Hong Kong, and he adapted it to his work now. His technique is pretty similar to the run for your life strategy, except his was to do the jumping jack which I'm going to show you later. He does this with his team and goes back to prepare for dinner right after their lunch break. I did not realized how powerful this technique was until I discovered it through a course I took a year ago.

Here are some situations we face that will cause stress:

- It's 5:50 P.M., you are *deciding/planning* what to eat or make for dinner is one of the most stressful time of the day.

- *Difficult or annoying* co-worker - We spend most of our working hours with them.

- Instead of going to the gym, you go to your children's school play.

- It's a nice day. You got out of work early to enjoy the rest of the day with family, but you are *stuck in traffic* because everyone was thinking of doing the same thing as you.

- You *couldn't sleep due to some unfinished work* at the office or an *important meeting in the morning.*

- Your boss asking for a *report that's past due* caused by someone else's negligence.

- One of your *children injured* him or herself at school, and you have to *rush to the hospital.*

- The *car broke down.*

- You kid *lost his or her new iPhone.*

- Your in-laws are coming over for the weekend.

- You are so *busy* that you don't have time to eat.

What do you do when you are *bombarded with so much stress, worries, self doubt and such stressful situations*? How do you let all the stress go and refocus? How do you come back to present and move and be productive? I would like to show you the fastest way to get out of a *head full of worries, self doubt, and irritability,* and to get back in focus.

Introducing run for your life:

Run For Your Life Strategy

Step 1

- Close your eyes.
- Notice the degree of stress that you have.

Then

Step 2

- Start running in place for 15 seconds as fast as you can.
- Run, run one, two, three.
- Keep going, keep running as fast as you can.
- Do not let anything distract you.
- Keep going, keep going.

And STOP

Step 3

- Now step back.
- Close your eyes and take a deep breath.
- Pay close attention to each and every one of your bodily sensations that move through you.
- Notice how it helps you bring your attention back.
- How it brings you into the present moment.
- When you go back to work, you will be more productive and less stressed.

This is the fastest way to reset your body when you are bombarded with stress, doubt, and worries. This strategy will bring blood flow throughout your body, bringing oxygen to the whole body to refresh your brain and mind and help you refocus and get back to productivity.

Your stress stops here! You can use any of the strategies in this book to help relieve stress. With the help of the mindfulness bell, or any reminder app, take a break to use these strategies every hour when you are at work or when you are in a stressful situation.

Bonus: Run For Your Life Strategy (Video)

Go ahead and **email your receipt from Amazon to the email below now** to see how it's done. Download *Your Stress Stops Here! Journal* so that you can keep a good record and see your progress.

Email your Amazon Receipt To:
join-stress@0s4.com

CHAPTER 9

Lift And Relax Strategy (Head Hold)

"Tension is who you think you should be.
Relaxation is who you are."

- Chinese proverb

The Jeweler

Stephanie owns a jewelry store in a hotel. She started out renting a booth in a jewelry store. She works really hard while raising her only son. Stephanie does her own *designs, creations,* and *picks her own stone*s carefully. She deals with all kinds of stones, ranging from jade, emerald, and sapphire, but mostly diamonds. She was the one who picked the stones for my wife's engagement ring. My wife, then fiancé, got together with her one day and together they designed and picked the diamonds for the engagement ring.

She came to me with a tight shoulder which she   thought

came from *sleeping on the wrong side* of the pillow, but told me that she has had the pain for quite some time. When I begin to get a feel of the area, I felt that it was more than just sleeping on the wrong side of the pillow. I asked her what position she sleeps on (sleep on the side, on the stomach, sleep with the hands up, sleep in a fetus position and sleep on the back), what her *work area* looks like, how she carries herself, how *she works* and how *she sits*. I took some mental notes while Stephanie was answering all the questions. She began to realize what she was doing at work that caused the pain.

We found out that *the chair* she was using *didn't support her back* and she spent most of her time sitting doing the designing, billing, and ordering. The only time she wasn't sitting was when she was out delivering or picking up her stones. *Her posture* contributed to her tense shoulders. She *hunched over* while looking at the diamonds and while *designing on the computer*. I suggested that to change her bed because it was old and not firm enough for her (she had the bed when her son was born; her son was fifteen years old at that time). I also told her to get a more *ergonomic chair*. I helped her loosen the neck, showed her how to sit and hold her *posture correctly,* and showed her the lift and relax strategy (shown below).

Veterinary Technician

Jane works as a veterinary technician at a very busy animal hospital in New York City. Jane is like a nurse to the animal kingdom. She gets in at 8 A.M. and starts getting her dental area ready by bringing in sheets, blankets, supplies, and turning on the machines. Once Jane is done setting up her area, she goes to the waiting room to admit her patients. She has to *take down their medical history*, make sure to take down any medication they are on, if any, and if the patient are seven years or older, they need X-rays and their owner needs to sign and agree.

After the paperwork and X-rays are done, the patients are moved to the waiting area where they wait patiently for their turn. When their turn is up, Jane has to premed the patient, carry the patient up the table (sometimes Jane has to assist the vet assistance to *carry big and heavy animal* to the surgery tables and then *carry them to post* surgery housing). She than has to put in the catheter, give them medication so they can get sleepy, and incubate the patient and start doing the surgery. After the procedure is done, Jane will wake her patient up, *move the patient* to a recovery room, and move to her next patient.

Jane moves on to *check on her in-hospital patients* after she finishes with all her dental patients. She administers injections and medication as per the vet's order when visiting the in-hospital patients every hour. She has to then help out in the outpatient area cleaning, medicating, and bandaging as part of wound care. She administers injections and medication, prepares patient by shaving the surgical area, prepares after surgery care, updates medical records, fills prescriptions and does blood work and urinalysis. At the end of the day, Jane *has to clean up*, mop her area, pack up the tools she used for the surgery, and set it to be sterilized. Some days, Jane has to *stay late* when there's an emergency, which happens at least three times a week. Her job is physically demanding, especially with the *carrying of the bigger animals* and the back to back schedule, all while also having to *wrestle with the patient that doesn't behave.* Constantly moving around adds more stress.

Optical Assistant/ Manager

Rebecca is an optical assistant /manager of an optical store. She has been working in this place for almost ten years and had worked herself up to management from just a clerk. She starts work at 10 A.M. and has to close up at 7 P.M. (sometimes later, depending on some late pick ups). She begins her day catching up with *paperwork, inputting customer's data and insurance information into the systems.*

She has to stop her data entry when a customer walks into the store. She'll show the customer what they ask for and also recommends glasses frames that she thinks are suitable for the customer, according to their price range. Once the customer has decided on the frame, the customer is sent to the optician for an eye examination. The customer comes back to Rebecca, and she'll *document the customer's history*, enter data into their health record, measure the eyes for the frame, set pick up glasses appointment, issue a bill, and accept payment. When the customer leaves, she has to make sure the frames and prescription are packed ready for their lab to be picked up by UPS. Rebecca's job also includes educating patients on glasses care and their service care when they come back to pick up their glasses, office upkeep (sometimes she has to clean the store's bathroom), *restocking inventory, filing claims,* and resolving customers' complaints. She sometimes has to go help the main store, which is five blocks away from her store. She goes to the main store to help out with *data entry* for insurance claims.

She spends many *hours on the computer*, and I noticed her neck and shoulder muscles were very tight. I asked her to describe her *work station* and the way she sits, the way she looks into the screen, the height of her chair, and her shoulder level when she's *working on the computer*. She told me that her *computer screen was non-adjustable* and her *shoulders* were close to her ears. She realized that sometimes she sits very close to the screen and felt the she *hunches* a little. I told her to ask her boss to have the computer screen changed to ease the strain on her neck. A few weeks later, her boss got her an adjustable screen.

During our time together, I helped her loosen her muscles, showed her how to sit properly *[Review Chapter 4 - Row Backwards Strategy, (Neck And Back)]*, showed her how her shoulders should be level with the neck, and also showed her the lift and relax strategy.

Ever woken up with a stiff neck? Slept on the side a little too often? Have you ever felt like pulling your neck out? Here is a simple tip to actually pull your neck, but not hurt yourself. You can do this strategy anywhere…whether you are at home, at work, in the subway, in the bus, playing tennis, after a bike ride…

Lift And Relax Strategy (Head Hold)

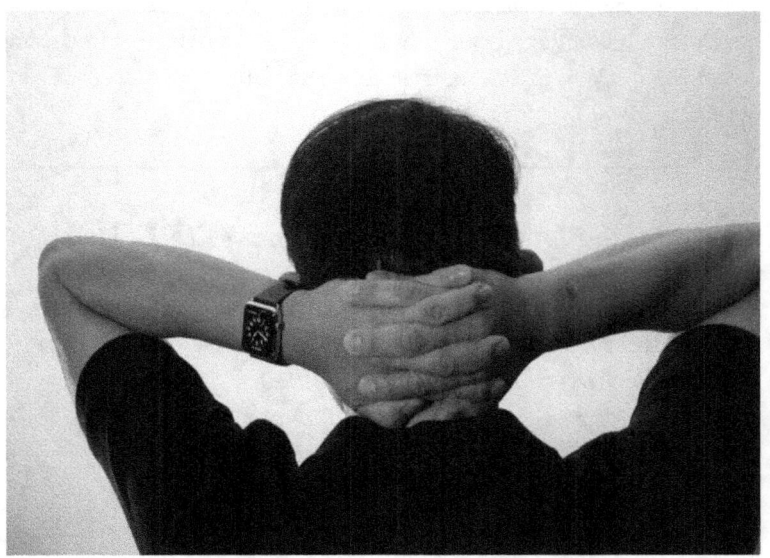

- Locate the right and left side of the bottom of your skull.

- Put your hands behind your neck.

- Fingers in between each other.

- Use the side of your hand, or the bottom of your palm, to lift the right and left sides of the skull.

- Breathe in and lift both sides of the skull when you exhale.

- Repeat three times.

As you lift the skull or the side of the skull, it begins to lengthen the neck, and you will feel the relief. You can use this strategy anywhere, as long as your hands are not holding anything!

Your stress stops here! You can use any of the strategies in this book at to help relieve stress. With the help of the mindfulness bell, or any reminder app, take a break to use these strategies every hour when you are at work or when you are in a stressful situation.

Bonus: Lift And Relax Strategy (VIDEO)

Go ahead and **email your receipt from Amazon to the email below now** to see how it's done. Download *Your Stress Stops Here! Journal* so that you can keep a good record and see your progress.

Email your Amazon Receipt To:
join-stress@0s4.com

CHAPTER 10

Breathing Away
Strategy (Stress)

*"Taking time out each day to relax and
renew is essential to living well."*

- Judith Hanson Lasater

Digital Graphic / Restaurant

Kenny owns a digital graphic company in New Jersey and recently started a restaurant in New York City.   Graphic design is his specialty, but cooking is his hobby. He is not the chef at the restaurant, but he oversees, plans and manages the restaurant. He spent the early half of the day with his graphic business after dropping his daughter to school, and the later half of the day was spent at the restaurant. Kenny *worked very hard* to establish his graphic business. He is very likable and is a gifted businessman. Over the years, he has built a large *network of people* in all walks of life. When he started the restaurant, it was   this group of people that supported him, and they are still supporting him by dining at the restaurant.

Kenny begins his day at 7 A.M., prepares breakfast for himself and his daughter. He goes into the office after dropping his daughter off at school at 7:45 A.M. He downloads the file that he finished a day before for printing and moves on with *his design work*. His work includes finish photo, mounting, set-up, and finishing touches. He also *delivers to his customers* and helps them set up. (A good example of customer service!)

He has to prepare to leave for the restaurant at 11 A.M. to help out with the *lunch hour rush*. After lunch, which is at about 2 P.M., he'll start up his computer and go back to his graphic work at his small office in the restaurant. He'll do his design and graphic work until 6 P.M., and then he has to prepare for the *dinner rush*. Kenny has to deliver food when the orders stack up and the delivery person is overwhelmed.

Kenny will move around from table to table to interact with his customers in the restaurant and also helps bring the food out. He likes to prepare decorative fruits for the customers. He really takes interest in his customers, and they enjoy his hospitality. He is usually at the restaurant until 10:30 P.M. He then *goes back to his office* to print out the work that he did at the restaurant. He has to do the mounting, framing, and get the order packed and *ready for delivery* or shipping.

He usually gets home around 2:30 A.M., falls asleep at 3 A.M., and gets up to do it again at 7 A.M. He gets an *extra few hours of sleep* only on weekends because he does not have to send his daughter to school.

You can imagine how much stress Kenny faces daily. First, *not getting enough sleep, the pressure from* running the two businesses, and lastly, the *daily travelling* between the company and restaurant is a *major stressor*. I remember him sharing with me that one of his mentors went to his restaurant to dine, and when he saw him doing all the work, told him that he *shouldn't be running* the restaurant, but should have someone running it for him. I can only help him by sharing the strategies in this book to help lessen his stress and hope that he will be able to find a trustworthy person to run the restaurant for him.

Garment Manufacturer

Chris owns a garment factory in Queens, New York. He and his wife run the company. Chris is in charge of bringing in the orders and drawing and cutting the patterns. His wife is responsible for the production side of the company. Chris lives in New Jersey, and him and his wife start their day at 5:30 A.M. They have to leave the house by 7 A.M. in order to *beat the rush hour traffic,* and usually get into the factory by 8 A.M.

When Chris gets an order from his customer, his wife Jane will write up a contract for the order. Once both sides agree with the order, Jane will start ordering fabric for the order. Chris will begin preparing for the pattern for the cutter to cut the fabric. Chris has to make sure the measurements are correct according to the sizes. His measurements must be accurate because it is important for him and the cutter to maximize the use of the fabric and prevent unnecessarily excess of non-usable fabric.

Meanwhile, Jane starts to set up a schedule working backwards from the delivery date. The absolute date to finish the order is a day before the shipping date. Jane then calculates the amount of garments needed to be finished. She also has to see if their factory could handle the workload or they need to subcontract out some of the work to other factories, but before she subcontracts out the order, she has to make sure the other factories are available to take the job. If there are not enough factories to help out with the order, Jane has to plan for extra amount of overtime to get the order done.

The cutting of the fabric begins when the fabric arrives and it is verified it's correct. The first sample is produced and sent to the customer for approval before production. As soon as the sample is approved, Jane and her team will start sewing, and the cut fabric will be shipped to the factories that will be helping with the order.

Chris will monitor the production of the other factories while Jane makes sure that her team is on schedule. In the garment industry, meeting the shipping date is very, very, very important because if the product wasn't shipped at   the contracted date, the customer can forfeit the factory by making the factory pay for their losses. This could take away a substantial amount out money from the factory, and could also determine if the company will make it or break it.

When all the sewing is done, Chris has to pick up all the finished garments from the other factories. Jane will lead her packaging crew with the packaging process for shipping. Jane takes a lot of time in planning the packaging process so that she can save time and money. She has to do this for every shipping because not all the packaging is the same.

Collecting money from the customers can sometimes be difficult and a little stressful. The fabric company usually wants their money 30 days after delivery. This creates a problem for Chris because he's under pressure by the fabric company to pay for the fabric they delivered, because sometimes his customers weren't able to pay him due to slow economy or for whatever their reason. This stress could be astronomical if they were working with two or more customers. It will definitely affect their cash flow and could possibly affect their workers.

I have shown Chris and Jane a breathing strategy that is very helpful and could be used anywhere, except while you're driving. This strategy is at the end of this chapter, and I want you to share your experience with this strategy in our private Facebook page.

Breathing The Pain Away

Relax your mind

Close your eyes

Step 1

- Inhale *deeply* through your nose right now.
- Exhale all the air flow out of your lungs.
- Just relax.

Do it one more time

Step 2

- Inhale through your nose.
- *Think about your shoulders relaxing.*
- Exhale all the air flow out slowly.

Step 3

- Inhale through your nose.
- *Think about your neck relaxing.*
- Exhale all the air flow out slowly.

Step 4

- Inhale through your nose.
- *Think about your upper back relaxing.*
- Exhale all the air flow out slowly.

Step 5

- Inhale through your nose.
- *Think about your lower back relaxing.*
- Exhale all the air flow out slowly.

Step 6

- Inhale through your nose.
- *Think about any area in your body that feels uncomfortable.*
- Exhale all the air flow out slowly.

Step 7

- Inhale through your nose.
- *Think about all your tension that may have built up.*
- Exhale all the air flow out slowly.

Now Focus On:

Step 8

- Inhale slowly.
- *Focus on releasing all your tension now.*
- Exhale slowly.

Step 9

- Inhale slowly.
- *Focus on releasing any emotion that you have built up inside you.*
- Exhale slowly.

Breathe in and breathe out as you relax deeper; know that you can let go of all the tension.

Step 10

- Inhale slowly.
- *Focus on letting go of all the anxiety and all the doubts.*
- Exhale slowly.

Take in a deep breath slowly, and as you breathe out, know that you can let go of all your anxiety and doubt.

As you do that, note that you are about to return back to what you were doing before, in a relaxed, stress free, and focused state of mind.

Your stress stops here! You can use any of the strategies in this book at to help relieve stress. With the help of the mindfulness bell, or any reminder app, take a break to use these strategies every hour when you are at work or when you are in a stressful situation.

Bonus: Breathe Strategy (VIDEO)

Go ahead and **email your receipt from Amazon to the email below now** to see how it's done. Download *Your Stress Stops Here! Journal* so that you can keep a good record and see your progress.

Email your Amazon Receipt To:
join-stress@0s4.com

CHAPTER 11

45⁰ 90⁰ And 135⁰ Strategy (Shoulder, Shoulder Blade)

"The time to relax is when you don't have time for it."

- Sydney J. Harris

Falco - Walking With God And A Dog

I was at a book writing seminar to learn about how to write this book out in San Diego, California when I met Andy Falco (author of *Falco - Walking With God And A Dog*.) Andy is a K9 (police) dog trainer and owner of the Falco K9 Academy in California. He recently closed a deal with the country of Bahrain to train all the country's police dogs because of his book. It was interesting to hear his story of how the Bahraini government found him as the number one bestseller with his five other books and contacted him for the deal. While we were talking, I noticed he was moving his shoulders and stretching his neck. I enjoy listening to his story, plus he was a fun person to be with. He asked me what I do, and I told him that I'm a massage therapist; I help people to de-stress and teach them simple techniques that they can follow to get rid of stress before it affects them. He gave me a big smile with a sigh of relief and asked me to check out his shoulder and neck.

The investigative side of me began to ask him questions as I began to palpate his shoulder and neck to look for tight or tense spots, sometimes called knots, which are caused by repetitive use of the muscle or stress on a group of muscles. At first, I was thinking life as a dog trainer shouldn't be stressful (like they showed on TV...all you need to do is make sounds like phssst, phssst and the dog will calm down and listen to your command). I came to find out that sometimes he has to carry or lift up the dogs he trains, and they vary in weight and also size. He's been doing these activities for many, many years. Over the years, he has accepted the stress on his shoulders and neck as part of life.

I found a few tight spots, or knots, in his shoulder blades and neck. When I worked on him, he felt currents running down his arm. He was enjoying my work while wondering why there were currents running down his arm. The current, according to Chinese or Eastern medicine, means there's a stuck Chi, or stuck energy, in the area. When I worked on it, the Chi, or energy, begins to flow again, thus the feeling of the current. The current gradually subsided, and I moved on to release the tension and the rest of the knots. He felt like a million bucks after I worked on him. I showed him the 45° 90° and 135° strategy (check it out at the end of this chapter) for him to do for maintaining this relaxation and preventing more stress.

ASK A QUESTION Section

I received a question from the "ASK A QUESTION" section of my blog from one of my readers.

Due to privacy policy, I'm going to call him Richard. Richard was asking for help with pain under his shoulder blade.

He said he found my videos on YouTube and went on to my blog. He said he had sudden pain under his left shoulder blade, and at first, he thought it was a torn trapezius. He googled and showed me the picture of the muscle under the shoulder blade. Richard felt pain when he lifted his arm up over his shoulder while at the same time leaning forward or sideways, and it was even painful when he coughed. He discovered that there was no pain if he pulled his shoulders back real tight to cough.

He said he couldn't think of anything specific, but he mentioned that he had been playing intense golf, but hadn't played for 10 years. He started playing a lot for the past three weeks. Now that he is hitting 50 years old in a couple of months, he is feeling the effects on his body. He also mentioned the he didn't have any medical, chiropractic, or physiotherapy help yet.

I asked him if he could point out where the pain was. Whether it was in middle left or upper right of the subscapularis (shoulder blade area) muscle base on the picture on the link he sent me.

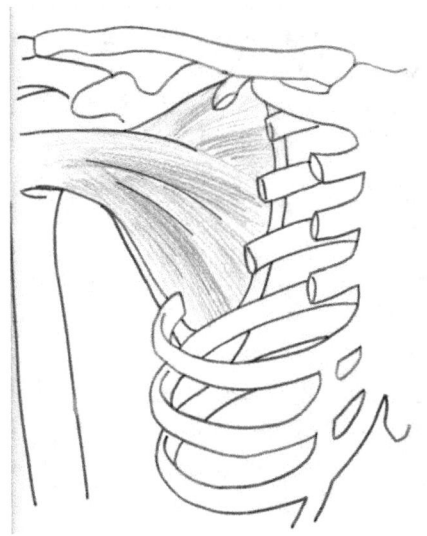

He said it felt like it was under the shoulder blade, but suspect that is was something else and sent me to a website. This site explained the symptoms of where he thinks the pain is. However, he can't really identify at which point he felt the pain - how should he go about locating the point? By pressing on it? How should it feel?

I'm going to show you three steps to shoulder blade relief.

Step 1

In order to locate where the pain is, you have to figure out what is a good muscle and what is a pain muscle.

How do you figure out what is a good muscle?

A stress muscle, a knot, or a tight muscle is call a stress or pain muscle.

How should a good muscle feel? For instance, touch an area on your arm or feel your thigh where there's no pain; just touch those areas, see how mushy it is, how bouncy it is. It's nice and soft; the muscle feels normal...no pain. That's a good, or pain free, muscle.

He said he had a pain on the left shoulder. So in order to compare to that, he has to press to feel the right shoulder and see if there's a difference. On the right shoulder, he should feel soft and mushy, nice and no pain, just like how we felt on the arm or on the thigh. On the pain area, you will feel tightness when you press on it; you will feel the pain.

Now we know the difference between a good muscle and a pain muscle, or tight muscle. When you work on it, you can feel how the tight muscle will slowly become soft muscle, and you can see and feel the difference.

Step 2

After locating where the pain muscle, tight spot, or knot is, I'm going to show you how to work on it.

- You go straight to the point or the area where the pain muscle, tight spot, or knot is, and put some pressure on it. Make sure you use the pads of your fingertips to press on the tight spot and then move your shoulders backwards, forwards, backwards, forwards, upwards and downwards.

- You move down to the next spot and repeat the same. Continue the same on all the spots, and you will feel the difference.

45° 90° and 135° strategy

- For this strategy, you need to find a corner of a wall, a doorway, a column, or even a lamp post. The 45° stretch will help relieve the lower part of the shoulder blade. The 90° stretch will help relieve the middle of the shoulder blade. The 135° stretch will help relieve the upper part of the shoulder blade.

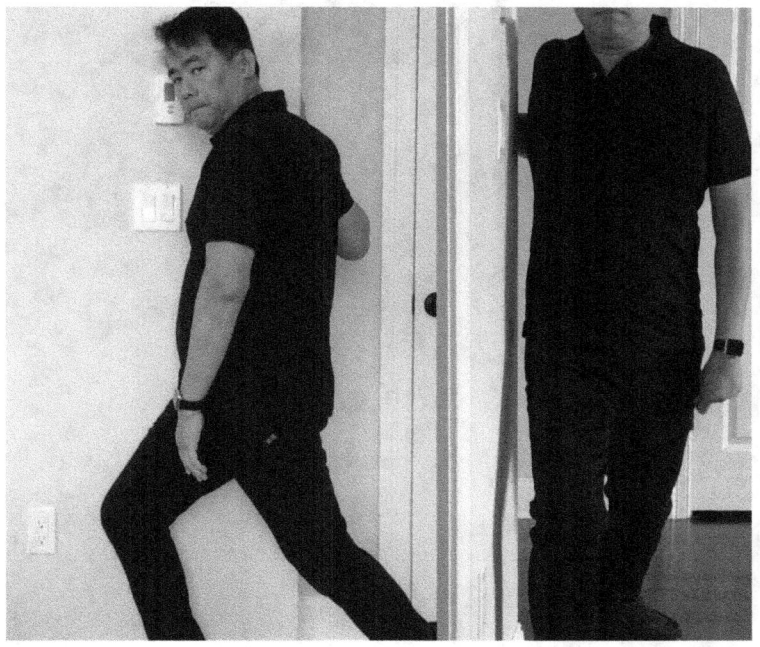

Same Hand Same Leg   *Front View*
(Body Close To The Wall)

45° Stretch relieves the **lower part of the shoulder blade.**

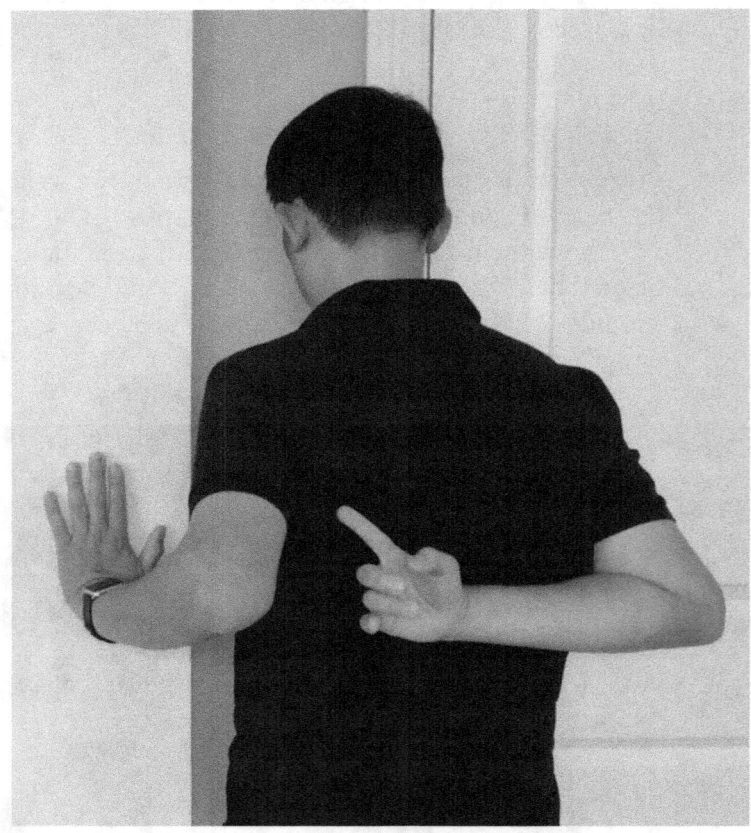

- Stand parallel to the corner of the wall or doorway.

- Put your hand at a 45° angle on the wall where the affected side, or the side where the pain muscle, tight spot, knot is.

- Take one step forward and bend your knee 90° (the affected side or the side where the pain muscle, tight spot, knot is).

- Just remember, same hand same knee.

90° Stretch relieve the **middle part of the shoulder blade.**

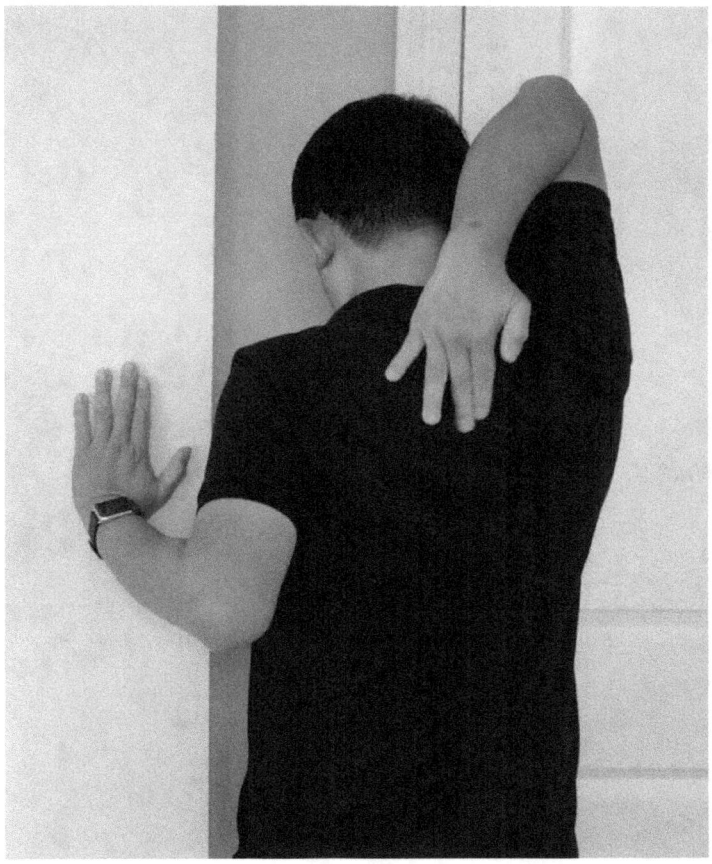

- Stand parallel to the corner of the wall or doorway.

- Put your hand at a 90° angle on the wall where the affected side, or the side where the pain muscle, tight spot, knot is.

- Take one step forward and bend your knee 90°(the affected side or the side where the pain muscle, tight spot, knot is).

- Just remember, same hand same knee.

135° Stretch relieve the **upper part of the shoulder blade.**

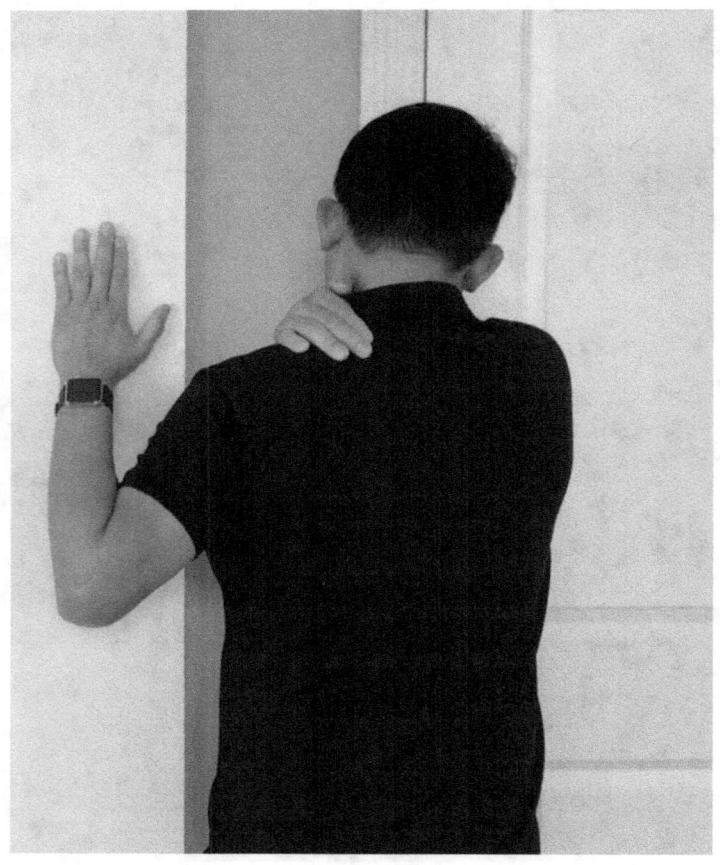

- Stand parallel to the corner of the wall or doorway.

- Put your hand at a 135° angle on the wall where the affected side, or the side where the pain muscle, tight spot, knot is.

- Take one step forward and bend your knee 90° (the affected side or the side where the pain muscle, tight spot, knot is).

- Just remember, same hand same knee.

45° 90° And 135° Strategy (Shoulder, Shoulder Blade)

You can use this strategy when you feel the tension, or the stress, building up, or when you are aware of any discomfort. This strategy is great for people who are on the computer a lot, who read a lot, carries baby, carries pets, or carries a heavy bag.

Your stress stops here! You can use any of the strategies in this book at to help relieve stress. With the help of the mindfulness bell, or any reminder app, take a break to use these strategies every hour when you are at work or when you are in a stressful situation.

Bonus:45° 90° And 135° Strategy (Video)

Go ahead and **email your receipt from Amazon to the email below now** to see how it's done. Download *Your Stress Stops Here! Journal* so that you can keep a good record and see your progress.

Email your Amazon Receipt To:
join-stress@0s4.com

CHAPTER 12

360° Slow Motion
Strategy (Neck)

"It's not stress that kills us,
it is our reaction to it"

- Hans Selye

It is no secret that working in an office can be quite stressful. An employee's biggest concern is the *amount of workload* being distributed to them. The constant acquisitions (bigger companies buying over smaller companies), or companies merging, cause employees to wonder if their job will be there if the company decides to consolidate the departments or even downsize. The thoughts of having an extra workload and having to *look for another job* make it more stressful for them.

There's one thing you, as an employee, have to understand - you are at a place of business and work needs to get done, and you get a paycheck for the work you do. You are there to make money for the owners, investors, or the stockholders. You need to know what your j*ob description* is and do what you are supposed to do. Check to see how you fit into the company and find out if there's room for growth. If the money you are earning is *not enough* to make ends meet, start looking for a better job. In the meantime, use your present job as a stepping stone to a bigger and better job. Knowing where you fit in the company will help you move towards positive stress.

Have you ever work through lunch and wondered why you were feeling so weak at the end of the work day? Do you know why lunch breaks and other breaks were created? Yes, it is for you to take a break from your work. Lunch break is the time for you to take in some food to replenish the energy burned during the day. When I was working in corporate America, employees were allowed to take cigarette smoke breaks several times a day. If they are allow to take a smoke break (not that I'm advocating smoking), non-smokers should also be allowed to take a break.

You can walk to your cafeteria for a bottle of water, some snacks, a bag of nuts or a cup of fruit. If you don't have a cafeteria, just step out of the office to the store nearby. The goal here is not to encourage you to be lazy, but to recharge you. There are multiple studies stating that employees who take breaks are *more productive* compared to those who don't. In the *Business Insider* article "Here's How Much Work Your Brain Can Handle Before Needing a Break," it shared a study conducted by the Draugiem Group. They found that, "people who were religious about taking short breaks were far more productive than those who worked longer hours.[13]" Turning away from work, or not thinking about work, allows you to put your attention to something else for a few minutes. This is a good *stress relief practice.*

When approaching crunch time, you need to prioritize your work according to its importance or try doing some of the work ahead of time. It is important to try NOT to bring work home.

---

[13] "Here's how much work your brain can handle before ..."
<http://www.businessinsider.com/this-is-the-perfect-amount-of-time-to-work-each-day-2016-1?pundits_only=0&get_all_comments=1&no_reply_filter=1>

WHY? Because work is work no matter how much you do, no matter how hard you work, IT'S going to be there. Like one of my mentors always says, "No one dies." It's alright if it's not done, only delayed. If you absolutely need to bring work home, try going to work earlier instead of bringing it home.

How to reduce physical stress? Some of your answers may be: deep breathing, meditating, being present, stretching, exercising, being grateful, getting outdoors, sharing with someone, laughing out loud, decluttering, journaling, and the list goes on. The best way to reduce physical stress is by moving the stressed part of your body in a super slow motion.

What do you normally do when you feel tension on your neck? Your answer may be to stretch the neck and shoulder by moving them around or ask your friend to massage it for you. Before I learned this strategy and before massage school, sometimes I would just hit the area with a little force because of the unbearable tension.

Try stretching your neck by rolling your head. I want you to take 5 seconds to roll your head slowly. No! no! no! You are rolling your neck a little too fast! Most people (just like me in the beginning) normally roll their head too quickly, and your brain can't process anything. Time to learn how it's done correctly.

360° Slow Motion Strategy

- I want you to take 59 seconds to move your head slowly to make a loop. It was very hard for me in the beginning because I was impatient and I'd learned to stretch by moving vigorously.

Caution: Do Not Do This when you are driving or operating any moving vehicle.

- It takes practice and patience to get it. Once you get it, you will feel how your body reacts as you slowly bring the blood flow back to your body and release the tense areas. By engaging your muscles and focusing on how your body feels, you'll be increasing awareness, and through that awareness, your brain will send relaxation signals to the muscle.

Do this strategy as often as you need because it doesn't require much! Record it down in **Your Stress Stops Here! Journal**

Your stress stops here! You can use any of the strategies in this book at to help relieve stress. With the help of the mindfulness bell, or any reminder app, take a break to use these strategies every hour when you are at work or when you are in a stressful situation.

Bonus: 360 Slow Motion Strategy (Video)

Go ahead and **email your receipt from Amazon to the email below now** to see how it's done. Download *Your Stress Stops Here! Journal* so that you can keep a good record and see your progress.

Email your Amazon Receipt To:
join-stress@0s4.com

Final Thoughts

"When we commit to action,
to actually doing something
rather than feeling trapped by events,
the stress in our life becomes manageable."

- Greg Anderson

My goal in writing this book was to show how stress can affect you during daily tasks. There are things that you do that you think are not important that could cause stress in your life. For example: not paying attention to your posture, either sitting or standing, or not getting proper treatment after an accident (you can clearly see that in Chapter 4 and 7).

Stress is going to be part of our lives no matter what happens. You can either let it control you or you can control it. The ten strategies that I shared with you, together with the mindfulness bell and any reminder apps, are tools that you can use to manage your stress. You can use only one strategy or use two or three of these strategies when reminded by the bell, or app, to take a break.

I hope that you are more aware of what stress can do to you and *know the symptoms* that are affecting your body.

I hope that these strategies and stories have given you a few ideas about how to *control your stress*.

I hope that you feel ready to take on the shoulder tightness when you spend too much time on the computer and know how to *properly adjust yourself to comfort*.

I hope that you will know how to *de-stress quickly and go right back to work stress-less*.

I hope that you start using these strategies daily and make it *part of your lifestyle*.

These strategies have been *personally tested and modify* by me from what I have learned from my client and mentors. I do not only *teach them, but I personally use them*.

I wish you - *Your Stress Stops Here!* And BE WELL!

Don't Forget To Claim Your Bonuses
Email your Amazon Receipt To:
join-stress@0s4.com

About The Author

Vincent is the founder and president of StressedOutStressFree.com, a site dedicated to helping people with stress at their workplace. His experience in the corporate workplace while attending massage school has helped him understand the need to overcome stress caused by the workplace.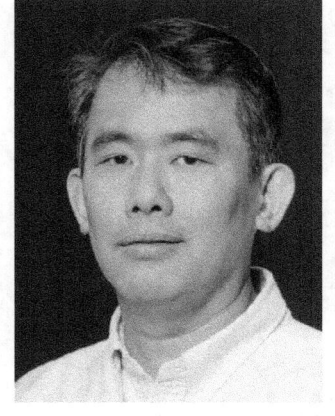

He helped launch a corporate massage program for a company in New York, working with the executives, secretaries, VPs, managers, janitors, IT people, salespeople, receptionists, and even the guards to help them release their stress.

His work with corporate massage has opened his eyes to the need to come up with a program to help people struggling with stress in their workplace. He created *Your Stress Stops Here* as a tool for them to figure out how to turn their stressful environment into a stress-less one.

His YouTube channel *StressedOutStressFree* has helped many people with their stress, tensions, and pain. His channel has over 3 million views at the time of this publication.

He loves food and travel. He will go the distance to acquire great food and beautiful places. He would drive five hours to

Maine from New York just for the lobster and enjoy the beaches there.

Learn more about how Vincent
can help you reduce your stress by visiting
StressedOutStressFree.com.